FOOD

&

MOOD

DIPAN KUMAR DAS
SUDIP KUMAR DAS

This book, "Food and Mood," is dedicated to all those who have embarked on a journey to understand the profound connection between what we eat and how we feel.

To the individuals who have courageously navigated the complex terrain of emotional well-being, may these pages serve as a source of inspiration and knowledge, empowering you to make informed choices for a happier, healthier life.

To the friends, families, and support systems that stand by our sides, offering love and encouragement in our pursuit of emotional balance, this dedication is a tribute to your unwavering support.

And to the researchers, scientists, and healthcare professionals who tirelessly work to unravel the mysteries of the food-mood connection, we extend our gratitude for your commitment to improving our understanding of this intricate relationship.

May this book shed light on the path to emotional resilience, offering hope and empowerment to all who seek a harmonious connection between food and mood.

Foreword

In the pages of "Food and Mood," you are about to embark on a remarkable journey—one that delves deep into the intricate relationship between what we eat and how we feel. This exploration is a testament to the profound connection between our dietary choices and our emotional well-being.

In a world where the significance of mental health is increasingly recognized, "Food and Mood" offers a comprehensive guide to understanding how the foods we consume can have a transformative impact on our emotions. It reveals the power we hold in our hands, and on our plates, to shape our emotional states and resilience.

This book is not just a collection of words; it is an invitation to a transformative experience. Within these chapters, you will discover the latest insights from the fields of nutrition, psychology, and neuroscience. You will explore personal narratives of those who have harnessed the power of mindful dietary choices to transform their emotional lives. You will gain a deeper understanding of how stress, anxiety, and depression are linked to what we eat, and how we can mitigate their effects through nutrition.

The journey through "Food and Mood" is not a one-way path; it is a conversation between the pages and your understanding, your choices, and your life. As you progress, you will find practical tools and actionable advice to help you make informed decisions about your diet and emotional well-being.

As the reader, you are at the helm of this exploration, and the choices you make as you read and reflect have the potential to ripple into your daily life, transforming your relationship with food and your emotional state.

This book is a tribute to the complexities of the human experience and a testament to our capacity for growth, resilience, and well-being. We invite you to join us in this exploration, to open your mind to new insights, and to empower yourself with the knowledge to make informed choices for a more emotionally balanced and resilient you.

Welcome to the transformative journey of "Food and Mood."

Preface

In an ever-evolving world, the intersection of food and mood has emerged as a frontier of understanding and empowerment. Our emotional well-being is a complex tapestry, woven from the threads of our thoughts, feelings, and experiences. Yet, hidden within this tapestry is the profound influence of the foods we choose to consume.

This book, "Food and Mood," is a journey into the heart of that influence. It is a testament to the power of nutrition to shape our emotional states and enhance our resilience in the face of life's challenges. Within these pages, we explore the fascinating connections between what we eat and how we feel, from the intricate dance of nutrients in our bodies to the ways in which our dietary choices can impact stress, anxiety, and depression.

"Food and Mood" is not just a collection of facts and figures. It is an invitation to a transformative experience, one that empowers you with the knowledge and tools to make informed choices for a happier, healthier emotional life. Throughout this book, you'll encounter the latest insights from the fields of nutrition, psychology, and neuroscience. You'll discover personal narratives of individuals who have harnessed the power of mindful dietary choices to transform their emotional lives. You'll gain a deeper understanding of the science behind the food-mood connection, and you'll find practical advice to help you make changes in your diet that support your emotional well-being.

As you turn the pages, you become an active participant in this exploration. The choices you make as a reader have the potential to ripple into your daily life, affecting not only what you eat but also how you experience and respond to your emotions. It is a journey of self-discovery, one that invites you to embrace the power you hold to shape your own emotional narrative.

Our hope is that "Food and Mood" will serve as a source of inspiration and empowerment, as well as a reminder that the journey to emotional resilience is one worth taking. We invite you to open your mind to new insights, to challenge your preconceptions, and to embrace the transformative potential of mindful dietary choices.

Welcome to the exploration of "Food and Mood."

Prologue

In the heart of every culture, food has been celebrated not only as sustenance for the body but also as a source of comfort, connection, and joy for the soul. Our relationship with food is deeply intertwined with our emotions, and throughout history, this connection has been acknowledged in the art of cooking, the rituals of feasting, and the sharing of meals with loved ones.

In the 21st century, our understanding of this age-old relationship has deepened. We now possess the knowledge, tools, and insights to explore the intricate interplay between what we eat and how we feel. This exploration is at the heart of "Food and Mood."

In the chapters that follow, you will embark on a journey into the world of nutrition, psychology, and neuroscience. You will delve into the science behind the food-mood connection, discovering how the nutrients we consume can influence our emotional well-being. You will hear personal narratives of individuals who have harnessed the power of mindful dietary choices to transform their emotional lives. And you will find practical advice to help you make informed decisions about your diet and emotional health.

This book is more than a collection of facts and figures; it is an invitation to a transformative experience. It is an acknowledgment of the power you hold in your hands, and on your plates, to shape your emotional states and enhance your resilience in the face of life's challenges.

The journey of "Food and Mood" is a dialogue, a conversation between the pages and your understanding, your choices, and your life. As you read and reflect, you become an active participant in this exploration, and the choices you make have the potential to ripple into your daily life, transforming your relationship with food and your emotional well-being.

It is a journey of self-discovery, one that invites you to embrace the power you hold to shape your own emotional narrative. Through this exploration, may you find inspiration, empowerment, and a deeper understanding of the profound connection between what you eat and how you feel.

Welcome to the transformative journey of "Food and Mood."

CHAPTER ONE

Introduction: The Food-Mood Connection

In a world where the pace of life seems to quicken with each passing day, and stress, anxiety, and mood disorders have become commonplace, the link between what we eat and how we feel is an increasingly pertinent subject of exploration. Welcome to "Food and Mood," a journey into the fascinating and often surprising interplay between the foods we consume and our emotional well-being.

Throughout history, our connection to food has transcended mere sustenance. We gather around tables to celebrate joyous occasions, share stories of our day over a meal, and seek solace in comfort foods when we're down. But what if this relationship with food runs even deeper than we imagined? What if the foods we choose can, in fact, be instrumental in shaping our emotional landscape, influencing our happiness, our stress levels, and even our mental health?

This book embarks on a quest to unlock the secrets of the food-mood connection. It's a journey that will take us through the realms of nutrition and psychology, delving into the intricate science of the gut-brain axis, the power of essential nutrients, and the subtle art of mindful eating. We will explore the ways in which our food choices can lift our spirits or plunge us into the depths of despair. We will confront the dark side of our modern diets, understanding how they can contribute to the rising tide of mental health challenges.

Yet, "Food and Mood" is not just a catalog of the problems; it's a guide to solutions. We'll uncover the culinary keys to happiness, offering you practical advice on how to leverage the foods you love to enhance your emotional well-being. From the foods that soothe stress to those that combat anxiety, we will unveil a treasure trove of dietary strategies that can empower you to take charge of your emotions.

But this book is more than just a compilation of facts and figures. It's a testament to the incredible interplay between the science of nutrition and the art of living well. As we embark on this journey, we will discover that the path to emotional balance is both a deeply personal and a universal quest. It's a path paved with the flavors, aromas, and textures of the foods we savor, but it's also a path lined with the science that demystifies their effects on our mood.

"Food and Mood" is an invitation to explore the profound connection between what's on your plate and how you feel. It's an exploration of the gut instincts that guide our dietary choices and the scientific insights that back them up. So, join us as we embark on a voyage through the intricate landscape of the food-mood connection, unlocking the doors to emotional well-being, one bite at a time.

This book is your compass for navigating the intricate world of food and mood, helping you make informed choices that not only fuel your body but also nurture your emotional health. As we delve into this exciting journey, you'll gain a deeper appreciation for the profound impact that your diet can have on your overall well-being.

As we explore the topics ahead, we'll discuss the science behind the food-mood connection. We'll examine the remarkable communication system known as the gut-brain axis, where the foods you consume can influence your emotions, and your emotional state can, in turn, impact your digestive system. We'll unravel the mystery of essential nutrients, those vital elements in your diet that play a fundamental role in maintaining emotional balance. And we'll also delve into the psychological aspects of eating, understanding how your emotions can drive your food choices and, conversely, how your food choices can shape your emotions.

But this book is not just a compendium of scientific studies and expert advice; it's also a practical guide for enhancing your emotional well-being through food. We'll explore specific foods and dietary habits that can boost your mood and alleviate stress, anxiety, and even depression. From the vibrant colors of fruits and vegetables to the soothing warmth of a cup of herbal tea, you'll discover a cornucopia of options for enhancing your mood.

The journey to a healthier, happier you begins here. It's an invitation to explore the wonderful world of food and mood, to embrace the idea that you have the power to influence your emotional well-being through your dietary choices. By the end of this book, you'll not only be armed with knowledge but also equipped with practical strategies to make better food choices for a brighter, more emotionally balanced future.

So, as we set forth on this voyage, I encourage you to approach it with an open mind and a willingness to make small, meaningful changes to your diet. The food-mood connection is a powerful and transformative concept, and by the time you reach the final chapter, you'll be equipped with the tools and insights to harness its potential in your life.

Buckle up and prepare to embark on a journey that will forever change the way you think about what you eat and how it makes you feel. "Food and Mood" is not just a book; it's an exploration of the profound and intricate relationship between what's on your plate and the emotions in your heart.

In the pages that follow, we will weave a narrative that intertwines science and sensibility, inviting you to connect with your food in a way that extends beyond mere sustenance. You'll learn how to nourish not only your body but also your mind and soul, embracing a holistic approach to well-being that acknowledges the deep-rooted connection between nutrition and emotions.

It's important to note that while this book provides valuable insights, it is not a replacement for professional medical or psychological advice. If you are struggling with severe emotional challenges or significant dietary issues, we strongly recommend seeking guidance from qualified healthcare professionals. This book should be seen as a companion on your journey to better understand and improve your relationship with food, offering practical tips and knowledge to complement your overall well-being.

Throughout our exploration of the food-mood connection, you'll find real-life stories, expert opinions, and practical exercises designed to empower you to make informed choices. You'll be equipped to distinguish between fleeting cravings and nourishing choices, and you'll gain a deeper appreciation for the mindfulness that can infuse your eating experiences. With the right tools and knowledge, you can cultivate a more positive relationship with food and, in turn, enhance your emotional state.

As we proceed through each chapter, you'll find an array of resources, recipes, and actionable steps to help you apply the knowledge you've gained. You'll also encounter thought-provoking questions and exercises that encourage self-reflection and personal growth. The journey through these pages is as much about understanding the food-mood connection as it is about understanding yourself.

This book is a roadmap to a healthier, happier you, one bite, one choice, and one emotion at a time. So, let's begin this adventure into the fascinating world of "Food and Mood." As we dive into the complex relationship between what we eat and how we feel, be prepared to be inspired, informed, and empowered to transform your life, one meal at a time. Together, we will uncover the secrets of emotional well-being hidden within the choices you make at your dining table, and we will set you on a path towards a more fulfilling and nourishing existence.

Now, let's embark on this journey, exploring the profound connections between the foods you choose and the emotions that shape your world. "Food and Mood" invites you to embrace a future where your dietary choices become not just a source of sustenance but a wellspring of emotional strength and vitality.

Exploring the Intriguing Relationship Between What We Eat and How We Feel

The connection between the food we consume and our emotional well-being is a journey of discovery that has fascinated scientists, health enthusiasts, and food lovers alike for centuries. From ancient wisdom to modern research, there is a growing understanding that the foods we choose to nourish our bodies can significantly influence our emotional state. This connection is not mere happenstance; it's a profound and intricate relationship that we are only beginning to unravel.

Consider a moment when you've savored a piece of rich, dark chocolate and felt an almost instantaneous sense of pleasure. Or think about how a warm bowl of chicken soup has the power to soothe not just a sore throat but also a troubled mind. These experiences are not coincidental. They are evidence of the profound impact of food on our mood, our emotions, and even our mental health.

As we embark on this journey of exploration, it's essential to recognize that the food-mood connection goes beyond the superficial. It's not just about feeling happy after indulging in your favorite treat or regretting the extra helping of comfort food. The relationship between food and mood is rooted in science, in the intricate workings of our bodies and minds.

In this introductory chapter, we'll take a closer look at the fundamental principles that underpin the food-mood connection. We'll delve into the idea that our bodies are complex ecosystems, and what we feed them has far-reaching consequences, extending well beyond our physical health.

The food-mood connection is, at its core, about the science of nutrition, the remarkable dialogue between our gut and our brain, and the powerful influence of essential nutrients. We'll explore how the choices you make at the dinner table can either nourish your emotional well-being or hinder it. It's a journey that promises to empower you with the knowledge and insights needed to make mindful, informed choices about your diet and, in turn, your emotional health.

Throughout this book, we will discover that the food-mood connection is a dynamic and ever-evolving field. It's a journey into the latest scientific findings, expert opinions, and practical advice that will equip you to take control of your emotional well-being through your food choices. The journey begins here, as we uncover the intriguing relationship between what we eat and how we feel, setting the stage for a transformational exploration of "Food and Mood."

CHAPTER TWO
Nutrition and Emotional Health

The intricate relationship between what we eat and how we feel is a topic of growing importance in today's fast-paced world. As we delve deeper into the nexus of food and mood, it becomes evident that the nutrients we consume play a vital role in shaping our emotional well-being. Chapter 2 of "Food and

Mood" embarks on a journey to unravel the profound connection between nutrition and our mental and emotional health.

The Building Blocks of Emotional Resilience

At the heart of this chapter is the idea that nutrition serves as the foundation for emotional resilience. Just as a house relies on a sturdy framework to withstand the elements, our emotional health depends on the nutrients that fuel our brains and bodies. In this section, we'll explore the role of essential nutrients in maintaining a stable and balanced emotional state.

Micronutrients and Mood: We'll delve into the impact of vitamins and minerals, such as B vitamins, vitamin D, and magnesium, on mood regulation. These micronutrients are the unsung heroes of emotional well-being, and understanding their significance is essential for a healthier, happier life.

Omega-3 Fatty Acids and the Brain: The role of omega-3 fatty acids in maintaining brain health is a central theme in this section. We'll explore their connection to mood disorders, such as depression and anxiety, and how incorporating them into your diet can promote emotional stability.

The Food-Mood Connection in Practice

This chapter is not just a theoretical exploration of nutrition and emotional health. We'll also offer practical advice on how to incorporate mood-boosting nutrients into your daily meals. You'll discover how to make dietary choices that support your mental well-being, whether it's through wholesome foods, supplements, or mindful eating practices.

A Personal Journey

Interspersed within this chapter are personal stories of individuals who have experienced significant improvements in their emotional health through dietary changes. Their journeys serve as a testament to the transformative power of nutrition on mood and emotional well-being.

Looking Ahead

As we wrap up our exploration of nutrition and emotional health, we'll foreshadow the chapters to come. The food-mood connection is a multifaceted subject, and we're just scratching the surface. In the chapters that follow, we'll delve into the complex science of the gut-brain axis, uncover the foods that can lift your spirits, and address the darker side of our modern diets.

So, as we conclude this chapter, consider the foods on your plate as more than just sustenance. They are the building blocks of emotional well-being, the catalysts for a happier, more balanced life. Join us as we continue to unearth the mysteries of the food-mood connection in the chapters that follow, and discover the empowering role you can play in shaping your emotional health through your dietary choices.

Mindful Eating for Emotional Well-being

One of the key takeaways from this chapter is the importance of mindful eating. It's not just about what you eat but how you eat. We'll explore the concept of mindful eating as a practice that not only enhances your connection to the food you consume but also promotes emotional well-being. Mindful eating encourages you to savor every bite, listen to your body's cues, and recognize the emotional triggers that can lead to unhealthy eating habits.

Eating Habits and Emotional Triggers: We'll discuss how certain emotional states can drive us to make poor dietary choices, leading to a cycle of emotional eating. By becoming more mindful of these triggers, you can break free from this cycle and make more intentional choices.

Sensory Pleasure and Emotional Satisfaction: In this section, we'll explore the sensory aspects of eating and how they contribute to emotional satisfaction. From the aroma of freshly baked bread to the vibrant colors of a salad, we'll uncover how these sensory experiences can enhance your mood.

The Role of Portion Control: We'll also delve into the importance of portion control in mindful eating. By understanding the right portion sizes for your body and being attuned to your satiety signals, you can maintain a healthy relationship with food and emotional health.

The Power of Hydration

In addition to the foods we consume, we'll also discuss the often-overlooked role of hydration in emotional health. Dehydration can lead to mood disturbances, and ensuring you drink an adequate amount of water is a simple yet effective way to support your emotional well-being.

Nourishing Your Brain and Your Emotions

Chapter 2 of "Food and Mood" aims to leave you with a sense of empowerment, recognizing that your dietary choices can significantly impact your emotional health. By nourishing your brain with essential nutrients, practicing mindful eating, and staying hydrated, you are taking the first steps towards a more emotionally balanced life.

As we conclude this chapter, we encourage you to reflect on your own dietary habits and their effects on your emotional state. How can you incorporate more mood-boosting nutrients into your meals? What changes can you make to practice mindful eating and savor the flavors and textures of your food more fully?

In the chapters that follow, we will continue to explore the complex web of the food-mood connection. The journey into the fascinating world of "Food and Mood" is far from over, and each chapter brings us closer to a more profound understanding of how the foods we choose can shape our emotional well-being. So, join us as we delve deeper into this transformative exploration of nutrition and its profound impact on our emotions.

CHAPTER THREE

The Gut-Brain Axis: Unravelling the Connection

As we journey deeper into the captivating relationship between what we eat and how we feel, we arrive at a critical juncture in our exploration—the gut-brain axis. In Chapter 3 of "Food and Mood," we embark on a fascinating voyage to understand this complex and dynamic connection between our digestive system and our emotions.

The Symphony of the Gut

Imagine your gut as the conductor of a grand symphony, orchestrating a harmonious interplay of trillions of microorganisms, cells, and neural pathways. This "second brain," as some call it, holds the key to understanding how the food you consume can directly impact your mood and mental well-being.

Microbiota and Mood: We'll begin by delving into the world of gut microbiota—the diverse community of microorganisms residing in your digestive tract. The balance and diversity of these tiny inhabitants have a significant influence on your emotional health. We'll explore the fascinating research that connects gut microbiota to mood disorders, such as anxiety and depression.

The Enteric Nervous System: We'll unravel the intricacies of the enteric nervous system, a network of neurons that governs the gut's operations. This system communicates bidirectionally with the central nervous system, playing a crucial role in how your gut and brain interact.

Neurotransmitters and Gut Health: We'll investigate the production of neurotransmitters like serotonin and dopamine in the gut and their profound influence on mood and emotions. These neurotransmitters, often associated with the brain, are intricately linked to the gut.

The Impact of Diet on the Gut-Brain Axis

This chapter is not solely about the science of the gut-brain axis but also about how your dietary choices can modulate this connection. We'll explore the foods and nutrients that support a healthy gut and, in turn, promote better emotional well-being.

Probiotics and Prebiotics: We'll discuss the role of probiotics and prebiotics in fostering a thriving gut microbiota. These substances are found in certain foods and supplements and can be used strategically to support a balanced gut environment.

Fiber and Gut Health: Dietary fiber, present in fruits, vegetables, and whole grains, is a powerful ally in maintaining a healthy gut. We'll explore how a fiber-rich diet can positively impact mood and emotional health.

Mindful Eating and the Gut-Brain Connection

As we conclude this chapter, we'll reiterate the importance of mindful eating in the context of the gut-brain axis. Mindful eating is not just about savoring flavors and textures; it's also about being attuned to how your food choices can impact your gut, and, by extension, your mood.

In the chapters that follow, we'll continue to dissect the multifaceted relationship between food and mood. By the time you reach the end of "Food and Mood," you'll have a comprehensive understanding of how the foods you choose influence not only your taste buds but also your emotions and mental health. The journey into the intriguing world of the gut-brain axis is a pivotal step in this transformative exploration, leading us to deeper insights and practical strategies for nurturing your emotional well-being through your diet.

The Emotional Landscape of the Gut

In this chapter, we'll also introduce the concept of "gut feelings." These visceral sensations are not mere metaphors; they are real physiological responses orchestrated by the gut-brain axis. Understanding the emotional signals that originate from your gut can provide valuable insights into your mood and well-being.

Emotional Responses and the Gut: We'll explore how the gut-brain axis can trigger emotional responses. From "butterflies in the stomach" to a "gut feeling," we'll uncover the science behind these sensations and how they relate to your emotional state.

Stress and the Gut: The relationship between stress and the gut-brain axis is a critical topic in this chapter. Chronic stress can disrupt the balance of gut microbiota and contribute to mood disorders. We'll delve into the mechanisms through which stress affects your gut and, consequently, your emotions.

Food Choices for a Healthy Gut-Brain Axis

As we venture further into this chapter, we'll provide practical guidance on how to make food choices that support a healthy gut-brain axis. You'll discover dietary strategies to promote a balanced gut environment, enhancing not only your digestive health but also your emotional well-being.

Fermented Foods: We'll highlight the benefits of incorporating fermented foods like yogurt, kimchi, and sauerkraut into your diet. These foods are rich in probiotics and can contribute to a thriving gut microbiota.

The Mediterranean Diet: We'll discuss the Mediterranean diet as an exemplary model of a diet that promotes both heart and gut health. Rich in fiber, fruits, vegetables, and healthy fats, this dietary pattern aligns with the principles of a healthy gut-brain axis.

Cultivating Mindful Eating for Gut Health

In this chapter, we'll reinforce the importance of mindful eating as a practice that enhances the gut-brain connection. When you approach your meals with intention and awareness, you can positively influence the messages exchanged between your gut and your brain.

The Promise of a Balanced Gut-Brain Axis

As we conclude this chapter, we invite you to reflect on your own dietary choices and how they may impact your gut-brain axis. The gut is not merely a passive part of your digestive system; it is a dynamic player in the emotional symphony of your life. By understanding and nourishing this intricate connection, you can take significant steps toward a more balanced, emotionally fulfilling existence.

CHAPTER FOUR

Eating for Happiness: Foods That Boost Your Mood

Our culinary journey through the intricate relationship between food and mood continues in Chapter 4, where we turn our focus toward the foods that have the remarkable ability to elevate our spirits and promote a sense of happiness. In this chapter, we explore the science behind these mood-boosting foods and how they can contribute to a more joyful and emotionally balanced life.

The Science of Mood-Boosting Foods

It's not just a matter of coincidence or personal preference; certain foods contain specific compounds that can directly impact your mood and emotional well-being. In this section, we'll delve into the science behind these mood-enhancing elements.

Serotonin-Boosting Foods: We'll explore foods rich in tryptophan, a precursor to serotonin, often referred to as the "feel-good" neurotransmitter. Discover how these foods can help increase serotonin levels in the brain and, in turn, promote a sense of happiness and well-being.

Folate and B Vitamins: Folate and other B vitamins are essential for mood regulation. We'll discuss how foods rich in these nutrients can support the production of mood-stabilizing chemicals in the brain.

Foods That Brighten Your Mood

The heart of this chapter is dedicated to introducing you to a wide array of foods that have the potential to enhance your mood and bring a sense of happiness to your daily life.

Dark Chocolate: Dive into the world of dark chocolate, a treat that not only satisfies your sweet tooth but also contains compounds that can trigger the release of endorphins and boost mood.

Berries: Discover the antioxidant-rich nature of berries, which can help reduce oxidative stress and inflammation in the brain, potentially leading to improved mood.

Leafy Greens: Green vegetables like spinach and kale are packed with nutrients that support optimal brain function and emotional well-being.

Omega-3 Rich Fish: We'll revisit the importance of omega-3 fatty acids, this time with a focus on fish sources like salmon, mackerel, and sardines. These foods can promote cognitive function and help alleviate symptoms of mood disorders.

Combining Foods for Maximum Impact

As we explore the mood-boosting potential of individual foods, we'll also discuss how combining these items in your meals can yield a synergistic effect, providing an extra layer of support for your emotional well-being.

Mindful Consumption for Enhanced Joy

In this chapter, we'll emphasize the importance of mindful eating, encouraging you to savor and appreciate the flavors and textures of these mood-enhancing foods. The act of eating mindfully can amplify the emotional benefits of these culinary delights.

A Taste of Happiness

As we conclude this chapter, we hope you'll leave with a sense of excitement about the possibilities that lie within your daily diet. The foods you choose have the power to shape your mood and bring happiness to your life. By incorporating these mood-boosting foods into your meals with mindfulness and intention, you can embark on a path to greater emotional well-being.

In the chapters that follow, we will continue to explore the multifaceted connection between food and mood. Whether it's uncovering the darker side of our modern diets, addressing emotional eating, or delving into the power of mindful eating, each section of "Food and Mood" adds a layer to our understanding of how the foods we choose can influence our emotional landscape. So, join us as we embark on this journey to embrace the joy and happiness that lies within the foods we love to eat.

A Balanced Approach to Mood-Boosting Foods

While the foods mentioned in this chapter have the potential to uplift your mood, it's important to remember that they are most effective when integrated into a well-rounded, balanced diet. A key takeaway is that you can weave these mood-enhancing ingredients into your daily meals, making them a consistent and enjoyable part of your dietary routine.

The Art of Recipe Creation

To make the most of these mood-boosting foods, we'll provide you with a collection of delicious and nourishing recipes that incorporate these ingredients. These recipes will not only satisfy your taste buds but also provide you with practical ways to include mood-enhancing foods in your daily culinary adventures.

The Role of Lifestyle Factors

In addition to dietary choices, lifestyle factors play a vital role in harnessing the power of food for emotional well-being. In this section, we'll discuss the importance of regular physical activity, adequate sleep, and stress management as complementary components of a holistic approach to maintaining a positive mood.

Personal Stories of Transformation

To inspire and connect with readers on a personal level, we will share stories of individuals who have experienced significant improvements in their emotional well-being by incorporating mood-boosting foods into their lives. These stories serve as a testament to the transformative potential of dietary changes.

The Promise of a Happier You

As we conclude this chapter, we invite you to reflect on the foods you consume and the potential they hold to bring joy and happiness to your life. By making conscious choices and incorporating mood-boosting foods into your daily routine, you have the power to enhance your emotional well-being.

Join us as we continue our journey through the intricate web of the food-mood connection. In the chapters that follow, we will delve into emotional eating, the impact of diet on stress, and the role of nutrition in managing mental health disorders. "Food and Mood" is not just a book; it's a roadmap to a happier, more emotionally balanced you, one meal at a time.

CHAPTER FIVE

The Dark Side: How Diet Affects Mental Health

In the complex relationship between food and mood, it's essential to address the darker side of our modern diets. Chapter 5 of "Food and Mood" delves into the profound impact of dietary choices on mental health, exploring how certain eating habits can contribute to mood disturbances and exacerbate mental health disorders.

The Modern Diet Dilemma

As we begin this chapter, we confront the realities of the modern Western diet. The prevalence of processed foods, high sugar consumption, and excessive saturated fats is a growing concern, and these dietary choices have been linked to various mental health issues.

The Sugar-Depression Connection: We'll explore the science behind the sugar-depression connection.

Excessive sugar intake can lead to mood swings, insulin resistance, and inflammation, all of which are detrimental to mental health.

Processed Foods and Mental Health: Highly processed foods often lack essential nutrients and are rich in additives and preservatives. We'll investigate how these foods can affect the brain and contribute to mood disorders.

Inflammation and Mental Health

This chapter also delves into the role of chronic inflammation in mental health disorders. A diet rich in inflammatory foods can fuel systemic inflammation, which has been linked to conditions like depression, anxiety, and even cognitive decline.

Anti-Inflammatory Diet: We'll introduce the concept of an anti-inflammatory diet, which focuses on foods that can help mitigate inflammation and potentially alleviate symptoms of mood disorders.

The Gut Microbiota and Mental Health

We revisit the gut-brain axis in this chapter to explore how an unhealthy diet can disrupt the delicate balance of gut microbiota and subsequently affect mental health. Dysbiosis, or an imbalance of gut bacteria, has been associated with conditions like depression and anxiety.

The Vicious Cycle: We'll discuss how an unhealthy diet can lead to changes in gut microbiota, which in turn can influence mood and exacerbate mental health issues. It's a feedback loop that underscores the significance of dietary choices.

The Impact of Nutrient Deficiencies

Nutrient deficiencies can be another consequence of a poor diet. In this section, we'll examine how a lack of essential nutrients like vitamins, minerals, and omega-3 fatty acids can contribute to mental health disorders.

The Path to Recovery

As we conclude this chapter, we'll discuss the path to recovery and how dietary changes can play a crucial role in improving mental health. We'll offer insights into adopting a more balanced and mindful diet to support emotional well-being and mental stability.

Personal Narratives

Throughout this chapter, we'll interweave personal narratives of individuals who have faced mental health challenges and have experienced improvements by making dietary changes. Their stories illustrate the transformative power of a balanced and nourishing diet in enhancing mental health.

Join us as we continue our exploration of the intricate connection between food and mood. In the chapters that follow, we'll delve into strategies for managing stress through diet, explore the relationship between food and anxiety, and investigate how nutrition can play a comprehensive role in coping with depression. "Food and Mood" is a comprehensive guide to understanding the multifaceted influence of diet on mental health, and by the end of this journey, you'll be equipped with the knowledge and strategies to make more informed choices for a happier, healthier you.

Strategies for a Healthier Mind and Diet

This chapter not only serves as a wake-up call to the potential dark side of our dietary choices but also as a roadmap to recovery and prevention. We'll provide practical strategies for making positive changes in your diet to support your mental health.

Mindful Eating and Mental Health: We'll emphasize the importance of mindful eating practices, which can help you gain better control over your food choices and cultivate a more positive relationship with what you eat.

Nutrient-Dense Foods: Discover the power of incorporating nutrient-dense foods into your diet. These foods are rich in vitamins, minerals, and antioxidants that can bolster your emotional well-being and protect your mental health.

The Emotional Toll of Dieting

In this section, we'll explore the emotional impact of restrictive diets, such as extreme calorie counting, fad diets, and severe food restrictions. We'll discuss how these practices can lead to mood disturbances and a negative relationship with food.

Seeking Professional Help

It's important to acknowledge that addressing severe mental health issues through dietary changes alone may not always be sufficient. We'll highlight the importance of seeking professional guidance and support when managing mental health disorders.

A Community of Support

As we conclude this chapter, we encourage you to recognize that you are not alone in your journey toward better mental health. There is a community of support, including healthcare professionals, mental health experts, and individuals who have experienced similar challenges. By reaching out and sharing your journey, you can take significant steps toward improved mental well-being.

CHAPTER SIX
Emotional Eating: Understanding the Triggers

Emotional eating is a common response to stress, sadness, anxiety, and a myriad of other emotions. In Chapter 6 of "Food and Mood," we delve into the intricate landscape of emotional eating, exploring its triggers, consequences, and strategies to regain control over our dietary choices when emotions run high.

The Emotional Eating Conundrum

Emotional eating is a phenomenon that many people grapple with, often without a full understanding of why they turn to food when their emotions surge. In this section, we aim to shed light on the complexities of emotional eating and why it is so prevalent.

Stress and Comfort: We'll explore how stress, one of the most common triggers for emotional eating, can drive individuals to seek comfort in food. The connection between stress and our dietary choices is deeply rooted in our biological and psychological responses.

The Vicious Cycle: Emotional eating can lead to weight gain and feelings of guilt and shame, which, in turn, can trigger more emotional eating. We'll investigate how this cycle perpetuates itself and contributes to emotional and physical distress.

Identifying Emotional Eating Triggers

Understanding emotional eating begins with recognizing the emotional triggers that lead to these behaviors. We'll discuss various emotional states and circumstances that can prompt individuals to turn to food for solace.

Boredom and Routine Eating: We'll delve into how boredom and mindless, routine eating can lead to emotional eating. These behaviors often stem from a lack of stimulation or an absence of fulfillment.

Loneliness and Isolation: Loneliness can be a potent trigger for emotional eating. We'll explore how food can serve as a substitute for social interaction and how this affects our dietary choices.

Mindful Eating for Emotional Resilience

In this chapter, we'll emphasize the importance of mindful eating as a tool to regain control over emotional eating. Mindful eating practices can help you become more attuned to your emotional triggers and develop healthier responses to them.

Recognizing Physical vs. Emotional Hunger: We'll discuss how to distinguish between physical hunger and emotional hunger, allowing you to respond to your body's needs more appropriately.

Savoring the Moment: Mindful eating encourages you to savor the flavors, textures, and aromas of your food, providing a more fulfilling and enjoyable experience that can counteract the impulse to eat emotionally.

Coping Strategies for Emotional Eating

This chapter also offers practical strategies to cope with emotional eating and break the cycle.

Alternative Coping Mechanisms: We'll explore alternative ways to manage emotions, such as exercise, creative activities, and relaxation techniques, which can replace emotional eating as a response to stress and other feelings.

Building Emotional Resilience: We'll discuss the importance of emotional resilience in managing emotional eating. Developing coping strategies that foster emotional well-being can provide a strong defense against the urge to eat emotionally.

Personal Stories of Transformation

Throughout this chapter, we'll share personal narratives of individuals who have struggled with emotional eating and have successfully overcome this challenge. Their stories serve as inspiration and a testament to the power of self-awareness and resilience.

Join us as we continue our exploration of the intricate connection between food and mood. In the chapters that follow, we'll investigate the impact of diet on anxiety, explore strategies for managing depression through dietary choices, and delve into the role of nutrition in enhancing overall mental health. "Food and Mood" is a comprehensive guide to understanding the multifaceted influence of food on our emotions, and by the end of this journey, you'll be equipped with the tools and knowledge to make informed choices for a more balanced and emotionally resilient you.

The Importance of Seeking Support

In the quest to overcome emotional eating, we must recognize that it's often challenging to go it alone. In this section, we'll emphasize the importance of seeking support from friends, family, or even a mental health professional. Sharing your struggles and triumphs with others can be a vital source of encouragement and guidance.

The Role of Self-Compassion

It's essential to remember that emotional eating is a common response to life's challenges. This chapter aims to alleviate feelings of guilt or self-blame and encourages self-compassion. By acknowledging that emotional eating is a shared experience and that setbacks are part of the journey, you can cultivate a more nurturing relationship with yourself.

Building Healthy Habits

As we conclude this chapter, we encourage you to reflect on your own emotional eating patterns and the triggers that lead to this behavior. By identifying these triggers and developing healthier responses, you can gradually build new, more constructive habits that support your emotional well-being.

CHAPTER SEVEN

Mindful Eating: A Path to Emotional Balance

In the intricate relationship between food and mood, the practice of mindful eating stands as a powerful tool for achieving emotional balance. Chapter 7 of "Food and Mood" is a deep dive into the transformative impact of mindful eating on our emotional well-being.

The Art of Mindful Eating

Mindful eating is not merely a dietary approach; it's a way of life. In this section, we explore the core principles of mindful eating, which are rooted in self-awareness, intention, and the cultivation of a positive relationship with food.

Awareness of the Present Moment: We'll delve into the importance of being fully present during your meals, free from distractions. Mindful eating encourages you to engage all your senses and savor each bite.

Listening to Your Body: We'll discuss the significance of tuning in to your body's hunger and satiety signals, allowing you to respond to its needs more appropriately.

Non-Judgmental Observation: Mindful eating fosters a non-judgmental attitude towards your food choices. This can reduce feelings of guilt or anxiety related to eating, promoting emotional balance.

Mindful Eating and Emotional Resilience

The practice of mindful eating can significantly contribute to emotional resilience. In this chapter, we'll explore the ways in which it can help you manage emotions and stress more effectively.

Stress Reduction: We'll discuss how mindful eating techniques can be harnessed to alleviate stress. By focusing on the present moment and adopting a non-judgmental attitude, you can experience a reduction in stress levels.

Emotional Regulation: Mindful eating can empower you to better understand your emotional triggers and develop healthier responses to them. By mindfully experiencing your emotions without judgment, you can achieve emotional balance.

Incorporating Mindful Eating into Your Life

In this section, we offer practical guidance on how to introduce mindful eating into your daily routine. We'll provide strategies for transitioning from mindless eating habits to mindful practices that can transform your relationship with food.

Starting with One Meal: We'll suggest starting small, perhaps with one meal a day, and gradually expanding your practice to encompass all your eating experiences.

Mindful Meal Planning: We'll discuss the role of meal planning and how it can support mindful eating by ensuring that you have nourishing, satisfying options readily available.

Mindful Snacking: We'll address the art of mindful snacking, emphasizing that even snacks can be an opportunity for mindfulness and emotional balance.

Personal Stories of Transformation

Throughout this chapter, we'll weave in personal narratives of individuals who have incorporated mindful eating into their lives and experienced remarkable transformations. These stories serve as inspiration and a testament to the potential of mindful eating in achieving emotional balance.

Join us as we continue our exploration of the intricate connection between food and mood. In the chapters that follow, we'll investigate the impact of diet on anxiety, explore strategies for managing depression through dietary choices, and uncover the role of nutrition in enhancing overall mental health. "Food and Mood" is a comprehensive guide to understanding the multifaceted influence of food on our emotions, and by the end of this transformative journey, you'll be equipped with the tools, knowledge, and support to make informed choices for a more emotionally balanced and resilient you.

The Mindful Eating Toolbox

To help you implement mindful eating in your life, we'll introduce you to a variety of techniques and tools that can enhance your practice:

Journaling: Keeping a food diary can help you track your eating habits, recognize emotional triggers, and gain insight into your relationship with food.

Guided Meditations: We'll explore guided mindfulness meditations that focus on eating. These exercises can help you cultivate a deeper connection with your food and your emotions.

Breath Awareness: Incorporating breath awareness techniques can serve as a powerful anchor for your mindfulness practice, allowing you to stay present during meals.

Mindful Eating in Everyday Life

In this section, we'll discuss how to integrate mindful eating into everyday situations, including social gatherings, restaurant dining, and busy workdays. We'll provide practical tips for maintaining your mindful eating practice regardless of the circumstances.

The Connection Between Mindful Eating and Emotional Well-being

As we conclude this chapter, it's essential to recognize that the practice of mindful eating is not just about the act of eating itself; it's about fostering emotional well-being. Mindful eating can help you develop a healthier relationship with food, reduce stress, and support emotional balance.

Join us as we continue our exploration of the intricate connection between food and mood. In the chapters that follow, we'll delve into the impact of diet on anxiety, explore strategies for managing depression through dietary choices, and uncover the role of nutrition in enhancing overall mental health. "Food and Mood" is not just a book; it's a guide to understanding the multifaceted influence of food on our emotions. By the end of this transformative journey, you'll be armed with the tools, knowledge, and support to make informed choices for a more emotionally balanced and resilient you.

CHAPTER EIGHT

Nutrition and Stress: Managing Life's Challenges

Stress is an inevitable part of life, and how we manage it can significantly impact our emotional well-being. In Chapter 8 of "Food and Mood," we explore the intricate connection between nutrition and stress, offering insights into how dietary choices can help us navigate life's challenges with resilience.

The Stress Response

Understanding the body's response to stress is the first step in managing it effectively. In this section, we'll delve into the physiological changes that occur when we experience stress and how nutrition plays a crucial role in mitigating its effects.

The Fight-or-Flight Response: We'll explore the body's primal reaction to stress and how it can lead to the release of stress hormones like cortisol and adrenaline.

Stress and Diet: We'll discuss how stress can influence our dietary choices, often leading to unhealthy eating habits. Stress-related overeating, cravings for comfort foods, and erratic meal patterns are common responses.

Nutrients for Stress Resilience

Certain nutrients are known to support the body's ability to cope with stress and maintain emotional balance. In this chapter, we'll examine these stress-busting nutrients and the foods that provide them.

B Vitamins: We'll highlight the role of B vitamins, particularly folate and B6, in regulating mood and supporting the nervous system. These vitamins can be found in whole grains, leafy greens, and legumes.

Magnesium: Magnesium is another essential nutrient for stress management. We'll explore how magnesium-rich foods like nuts, seeds, and dark chocolate can help calm the nervous system.

Antioxidants: We'll discuss how antioxidants found in fruits and vegetables can help combat the oxidative stress that often accompanies chronic stress.

The Role of Hydration

In this chapter, we'll emphasize the importance of staying well-hydrated as a foundational element of stress management. Dehydration can exacerbate stress symptoms, so maintaining adequate fluid intake is crucial.

Stress-Reducing Foods

We'll introduce a selection of foods known for their stress-reducing properties. These foods can help you maintain emotional balance and cope with the challenges of daily life.

Green Tea: Green tea contains the amino acid L-theanine, which has a calming effect on the brain and can help reduce stress and anxiety.

Complex Carbohydrates: We'll explore the benefits of complex carbohydrates, found in foods like whole grains and legumes, in promoting the production of serotonin, a neurotransmitter that supports mood.

Meal Planning for Stress Resilience

Practical strategies for meal planning will be discussed in this section, emphasizing how you can structure your diet to support stress resilience.

Balanced Meals: We'll provide guidance on creating balanced meals that include a variety of nutrients to support your body's response to stress.

Snacking for Stress: We'll discuss how mindful snacking can help stabilize blood sugar levels and provide steady energy, reducing the potential for stress-induced mood swings.

Personal Narratives

Throughout this chapter, we'll share personal stories of individuals who have experienced the transformative power of nutrition in managing stress. These stories serve as real-world examples of how dietary choices can contribute to emotional balance in the face of life's challenges.

The Stress-Reducing Lifestyle

In addition to dietary choices, we'll emphasize the role of a holistic approach to stress management. This includes regular physical activity, quality sleep, and relaxation techniques as essential components of a balanced and resilient lifestyle.

Exercise for Stress Relief: Regular physical activity can help reduce stress and promote the release of endorphins, the body's natural mood lifters.

Restorative Sleep: We'll discuss the importance of quality sleep in stress management. A well-rested mind and body are better equipped to cope with life's challenges.

Stress Reduction Techniques: We'll explore stress reduction practices like meditation, yoga, and deep breathing exercises, all of which can enhance emotional well-being.

Seeking Professional Help

It's essential to acknowledge that severe and chronic stress may require professional intervention. We'll emphasize the importance of seeking help from a healthcare provider or mental health specialist if stress becomes overwhelming.

Building Resilience

As we conclude this chapter, we invite you to reflect on your own relationship with stress and how nutrition, along with lifestyle factors, can support your emotional resilience. By incorporating stress-reducing foods and practices into your daily life, you can develop the tools to better manage stress and maintain emotional balance.

CHAPTER NINE

Depression and Diet: A Comprehensive Approach

Depression is a pervasive and complex mental health condition that can significantly impact one's quality of life. In Chapter 9 of "Food and

Mood," we explore the intricate connection between depression and diet, offering a comprehensive approach to managing and potentially alleviating the symptoms of depression through nutritional choices.

Understanding Depression

Before delving into the dietary aspect, it's crucial to develop a clear understanding of depression as a mental health condition. In this section, we'll explore the various forms of depression, the symptoms, and the factors that can contribute to its development.

Types of Depression: We'll discuss different types of depression, including major depressive disorder, persistent depressive disorder (dysthymia), and bipolar disorder.

Symptoms and Impact: We'll delve into the symptoms of depression and the ways it can affect one's daily life, including emotions, relationships, and overall well-being.

Depression and Nutrition

The relationship between depression and nutrition is multifaceted. In this chapter, we'll explore the dietary factors that can contribute to the development or management of depression.

Inflammatory Diet: We'll discuss how an inflammatory diet, characterized by excessive sugar, saturated fats, and processed foods, can fuel inflammation in the body and contribute to depressive symptoms.

Nutrient Deficiencies: Certain nutrient deficiencies, including those of vitamin D, B vitamins, and omega-3 fatty acids, can impact mood and have been linked to depression.

The Gut-Brain Axis in Depression: We'll revisit the gut-brain axis to examine how imbalances in gut microbiota can be associated with depression and how dietary choices can influence this relationship.

Anti-Depressant Foods

In this section, we'll introduce a selection of foods that are associated with potential mood-lifting and anti-depressant effects. These foods can form the basis of a diet aimed at managing depression.

Omega-3 Rich Foods: We'll emphasize the importance of including omega-3 fatty acids in your diet, particularly from sources like fatty fish, flaxseeds, and walnuts.

Serotonin-Promoting Foods: We'll explore foods rich in tryptophan, which is a precursor to serotonin, and discuss how they can support mood.

Fruits and Vegetables: Antioxidant-rich fruits and vegetables can help combat oxidative stress and inflammation, which are often linked to depression.

Meal Planning for Depression Management

We'll offer practical guidance on meal planning and structuring your diet to support depression management.

Balanced Nutrition: We'll discuss the importance of balanced meals that provide a variety of nutrients to support mental health.

Mindful Eating: Mindful eating practices can help individuals with depression develop a healthier relationship with food and a more positive experience of meals.

Personal Narratives

Throughout this chapter, we'll share personal stories of individuals who have managed or coped with depression through dietary changes and holistic approaches. These stories serve as inspiration and a testament to the potential of nutrition in managing depression.

The Importance of Professional Guidance

While dietary changes can play a significant role in managing depression, it's essential to acknowledge that severe or persistent depression may require professional intervention. In this section, we emphasize the importance of consulting with a healthcare provider or mental health specialist to develop a comprehensive treatment plan that may include therapy, medication, and dietary adjustments.

Building a Support System

Managing depression often requires the support of friends, family, or a support group. In this section, we discuss the importance of building a strong support system to help you cope with the challenges of depression. Sharing your journey with others who understand can be a source of encouragement and strength.

Developing Resilience

In the final part of this chapter, we encourage you to reflect on your relationship with depression and how nutrition, along with lifestyle and therapeutic factors, can contribute to your emotional resilience. By incorporating anti-depressant foods and holistic approaches into your daily life, you can develop the tools to better manage depression and work toward emotional balance.

CHAPTER TEN

Anxiety and Food: Finding Calm in Your Kitchen

Anxiety is a prevalent mental health condition that can manifest in various forms, from generalized anxiety to specific phobias. In Chapter 10 of "Food and Mood," we explore the relationship between anxiety and diet, offering strategies for finding calm in your kitchen through mindful dietary choices.

Understanding Anxiety

Before addressing the role of diet in anxiety management, it's essential to develop a clear understanding of anxiety as a mental health condition. In this section, we'll explore the different types of anxiety disorders, their symptoms, and the factors that can contribute to their development.

Types of Anxiety Disorders: We'll discuss various anxiety disorders, including generalized anxiety disorder (GAD), social anxiety disorder, and panic disorder.

Symptoms and Impact: We'll delve into the common symptoms of anxiety and how it can affect daily life, relationships, and overall emotional well-being.

Anxiety and Nutrition

The relationship between anxiety and nutrition is multifaceted. In this chapter, we'll explore the dietary factors that can contribute to the development or management of anxiety.

Caffeine and Anxiety: We'll discuss how excessive caffeine consumption can exacerbate anxiety symptoms, leading to increased restlessness and nervousness.

Sugar and Anxiety: The impact of high sugar intake on anxiety symptoms will also be explored. Blood sugar spikes and crashes can contribute to feelings of irritability and anxiety.

The Gut-Brain Axis in Anxiety: We'll revisit the gut-brain axis to examine how an imbalance in gut microbiota can be associated with anxiety and how dietary choices can influence this relationship.

Anxiety-Reducing Foods

In this section, we'll introduce a selection of foods that are associated with potential anxiety-reducing effects. These foods can form the basis of a diet aimed at managing anxiety.

Foods Rich in Magnesium: We'll emphasize the importance of including magnesium-rich foods like leafy greens, nuts, and seeds in your diet. Magnesium plays a crucial role in calming the nervous system.

Chamomile and Herbal Teas: We'll explore the calming properties of herbal teas like chamomile and how they can help alleviate anxiety symptoms.

Fermented Foods: Probiotic-rich fermented foods like yogurt and kefir can support gut health and potentially contribute to reduced anxiety.

Meal Planning for Anxiety Management

We'll provide practical guidance on meal planning to structure your diet in a way that supports anxiety management.

Balanced Nutrition: We'll discuss the importance of balanced meals that provide essential nutrients for overall emotional well-being.

Mindful Eating Practices: Mindful eating can help individuals with anxiety develop a healthier relationship with food, reduce overeating, and alleviate anxiety-induced symptoms.

Personal Narratives

Throughout this chapter, we'll share personal stories of individuals who have managed or coped with anxiety through dietary changes and holistic approaches. These stories serve as inspiration and a testament to the potential of nutrition in managing anxiety.

The Importance of Professional Help

For individuals with severe or persistent anxiety, seeking professional help is crucial. In this section, we emphasize the importance of consulting with a healthcare provider or mental health specialist to develop a comprehensive treatment plan that may include therapy, medication, and dietary adjustments.

Building a Supportive Environment

Incorporating dietary changes to manage anxiety often requires a supportive environment. In this section, we discuss the significance of creating an environment that encourages mindful eating and supports emotional well-being.

Developing Emotional Resilience

In the final part of this chapter, we invite you to reflect on your relationship with anxiety and how nutrition, along with lifestyle and therapeutic factors, can contribute to emotional resilience. By incorporating anxiety-reducing foods and holistic approaches into your daily life, you can develop the tools to better manage anxiety and work toward a calmer and more emotionally balanced you.

CHAPTER ELEVEN

The Future of Food and Mood: Trends and Promising Research

As we near the conclusion of "Food and Mood," we turn our attention to the evolving landscape of food and its influence on our emotional well-being. Chapter 11 explores the exciting trends and promising research that offer new insights into the future of food and mood.

The Evolving Role of Nutrition

Nutrition's role in mental health is continually evolving, and the future promises groundbreaking discoveries and advancements in our understanding of how food affects our emotional well-being. In this section, we'll discuss the evolving role of nutrition in mental health and its potential to revolutionize how we approach emotional wellness.

Emerging Nutritional Trends

New dietary trends and approaches are emerging, driven by an increased awareness of the food-mood connection. We'll explore some of these trends and their potential to reshape our dietary choices and their impact on emotional balance.

Functional Foods: The rise of functional foods, fortified with nutrients to support specific aspects of mental health, is an exciting development. We'll discuss the potential of these foods to offer targeted emotional support.

Personalized Nutrition: Advances in personalized nutrition are enabling individuals to tailor their diets to their unique nutritional needs, potentially enhancing emotional well-being.

Cutting-Edge Research

In this section, we'll delve into cutting-edge research that is shedding new light on the complex interplay between food and mood. We'll explore the latest findings in areas such as nutrigenomics, the microbiome, and the gut-brain axis, all of which are contributing to a deeper understanding of how dietary choices impact our emotional health.

The Influence of Technology

Advancements in technology are transforming how we approach nutrition and mental health. We'll discuss how smartphone apps, wearables, and telehealth services are making it easier for individuals to monitor their dietary choices and emotional well-being, providing valuable tools for self-improvement.

A Holistic Approach

The future of food and mood embraces a holistic perspective, recognizing that emotional well-being is influenced not only by what we eat but also by our lifestyle, environment, and social connections. We'll explore the importance of a holistic approach to emotional wellness that incorporates nutrition, physical activity, mental health, and community support.

The Ongoing Journey

As we conclude this chapter and our exploration of the connection between food and mood, we emphasize that this journey is ongoing. The relationship between what we eat and how we feel is a dynamic field, continually evolving as science and understanding advance. By staying informed and embracing the principles of mindful eating, balanced nutrition, and emotional resilience, we can navigate this complex relationship with confidence and hope for a happier, healthier future.

Join us as we celebrate the future of food and mood and its transformative potential. This chapter marks the end of our journey, but it's also the beginning of your own exploration of how food can shape your emotional well-being. "Food and Mood" is not just a book; it's a guide to understanding the multifaceted influence of food on our emotions. By the end of this transformative journey, you'll be armed with the tools, knowledge, and support to make informed choices for a more emotionally balanced and resilient you.

Empowering Yourself

As we embark on the future of food and mood, it's essential to acknowledge the power you hold in your dietary choices. With the wealth of knowledge and resources available, you have the ability to make informed decisions that can positively impact your emotional well-being. In this section, we encourage you to empower yourself with the understanding that you can shape your emotional health through the foods you choose.

Spreading Awareness

Promoting awareness about the food-mood connection is an integral part of the future of emotional well-being. We encourage you to share the knowledge you've gained from "Food and Mood" with your friends, family, and communities. By spreading awareness, you can help others make informed dietary choices and improve their emotional health.

The Ongoing Journey

In the final words of this chapter and the book, we reiterate that the journey of understanding the connection between food and mood is ongoing. New research, emerging trends, and evolving technologies will continue to shape this field. As you move forward, remember that you have the knowledge and tools to adapt to the ever-changing landscape of food and mood, and to make choices that support your emotional well-being.

"Food and Mood" has been a transformative journey, equipping you with the insights and understanding to make informed choices for a more emotionally balanced and resilient you. As you embrace the future of food and mood, may you find continued inspiration and empowerment in the complex yet beautiful relationship between what you eat and how you feel.

Epilogue

In the pages of "Food and Mood," you have embarked on a transformative journey—one that delves deep into the intricate relationship between what we eat and how we feel. It's a journey that has explored the profound influence of nutrition on our emotional well-being, from the fascinating science behind the food-mood connection to the inspiring personal narratives of those who have harnessed the power of mindful dietary choices to transform their emotional lives.

As you reach the conclusion of this book, it's important to remember that this journey is not a one-time endeavor; it is a continuous exploration. The relationship between food and mood is dynamic and ever-evolving, as new research, emerging trends, and evolving technologies shape this field. Your journey toward emotional resilience doesn't end here; it continues into the choices you make daily.

Throughout "Food and Mood," you have gained insights, tools, and knowledge that empower you to make informed choices for a more emotionally balanced and resilient you. You hold in your hands the power to shape your emotional narrative through your dietary choices.

This book is not merely a collection of words; it is an invitation to a transformative experience. It is a celebration of the complexities of the human experience and a testament to our capacity for growth, resilience, and well-being. As you move forward, remember that you are the protagonist of this exploration, and the choices you make have the potential to ripple into your daily life, transforming your relationship with food and your emotional well-being.

The journey through "Food and Mood" is a conversation between the pages and your understanding, your choices, and your life. It is an exploration that invites you to open your mind to new insights, challenge preconceptions, and embrace the transformative potential of mindful dietary choices.

May you find continued inspiration and empowerment in the complex yet beautiful relationship between what you eat and how you feel. The path to emotional resilience is an ongoing one, and we encourage you to embrace it with hope and confidence.

Welcome to the next chapter of your journey—a journey of self-discovery, empowerment, and well-being.

.....***.....